STUTTER FREE

ASH #SHORTS

ANSHUMAN SHARMA

Made with ♥ on the Notion Press Platform
www.notionpress.com

To all the winners who would defeat stammering to win their right to speak without the fear of words.

Contents

Preface

Can you defeat stuttering be defeated to become a good speaker? The answer is YES. Stammering will be defeated to make you reach the pinnacle of success if you believe in yourself and are ready to put in the required efforts.

How will this happen? Stammering is due to anxiety triggered by the psychological fear of letters and words. It means that your subconscious mind has accepted the fact that you will not be able to speak a specific letter or word. It becomes a belief, making it real. You stammer. If you get rid of this faulty thinking from your subconscious mind, then your anxiety would diminish automatically to make you a better speaker without speech impediments. Note the following points:

- Stammering is a habit,
- It is triggered automatically,
- The problem of stammering can be solved by getting freedom from faulty habits.

We will share the main ideas, exercises and techniques of the people who have successfully defeated their stammering in the past and become good speakers with professional success and satisfaction.

It is said that stammering is a rigid habit that does not easily leave a person. Stories abound about the years of struggle with stammering without results. Even if the intensity of stammering is reduced slightly, it tends to bounce back even harder. After several failed efforts people accept their fate of living a life with a speech handicap.

We do not guarantee that everyone following this book will be able to cure their stammering completely. The main objective is to present exercises, techniques and ideas which have worked for other people and were responsible for developing their communication skills and personality and helping them to defeat their stammering to a certain extent. In some cases, stammering was cured to 99% while in other cases it was 70%, 75%, 85%, 92% and so on. This journey is going to be long and hard. The stammering is not going to be cured immediately or show any signs of abating for several months. But if the efforts are consistent and hard, the stammering would slowly weaken and start to loosen its grip on the person.

This is the fundamental objective of this book. We hope that many people around the world would benefit from this collection of ideas and techniques.

If you want to fight your stammering with full force, this book will stand with you in your struggle. If you have high expectations from yourself and believe that you will be able to defeat your psychological fear of stammering, then let us start the journey to better speaking without speech handicap.

CHAPTER ONE

Fundamentals

The Source of Ideas

We understand the problems faced by the people who stammer or parents facing the challenge of kids' stammering. The frustration to express themselves or the failure to communicate their message to others is limiting and debilitating.

Many people make fun of people who stammer while others show pity or sympathy. None of these is uplifting for the person who is fighting the battle for normal communication. It is also deeply troubling for the people associated with that person. That is the reason most of the people who stammer struggle to live a normal life. Many people lose their confidence and start to feel defeated. They tend to develop an inferiority complex which also affects their other activities in life and work. A person with the potential of becoming an entrepreneur, a politician, a researcher or a salesperson is unable to reach his true potential. It is loose-loose for all.

In most cases, stammering is the psychological fear of producing specific sounds or speaking specific letters or words. It could also be due to anxiety for some reason or unnatural breathing patterns. Whatever be the reason, the person starts to believe that he would not be able to speak properly and utter some words. This soon becomes a reality for him. With every instance of stammering, the psychological fear of words increases. Many people try to fight their stammering by taking medicines, visiting speech therapists and implementing weird suggestions of people. This keeps happening till the person stops trying and accepts stammering as his fate.

We need to understand that stammering for most people is just a hard behavior that refuses to go. At a certain point, it does not strengthen but it stays there. Different people would have different levels of stammering, that is their point of stammering saturation. The problem with this level is that it becomes a part of the life of the person. His mind and body accept it as normal and natural. They do not fight against it. That is a point when stammering makes its temporary home permanent.

Disease? No, Habit? Yes

Many people believe that stammering is a disease. This thinking varies based on regions, countries and cultures. In a few places, it is considered repulsive, while in other places people are more tolerant of stammering. It can be considered as a habit, a speech problem, a lack of confidence or a disease. If it is taken as a disease then it gets into all sorts of complexities of diagnosis, testing, medication and in some cases, surgery. All the pain endured to find the cure does not guarantee alleviation of the disease, instead, for a few cases, it may lead to even more complexities.

Ayurvedic or Homeopathic medication will not lead to negative side effects, but nothing guarantee success. Nothing can, as stammering is not a disease but instead a habit. If simply taking medication or going through an operating procedure would have solved the problem, then most of the people with stammering or their families would have opted for it. But something must be done to solve the problem.

As discussed later that except in a few cases of stammering, which can be considered the cases of neurological stammering, most cases of stammering are developmental stammering, the stammering which begins in our developmental phase during childhood. This simple speech problem develops into a rigid and automatic habit of developing stress during speaking, which is difficult to break.

We do not consider stammering a disease but instead a habit that has been transformed into a rigid behavior, that is triggered automatically. We will try to weaken and break this habit by using self-managed exercises, techniques and ideas. We will not be using any type of medication or operating procedures to change the natural state of the body. Our approach would be different from procedures suggested or used by many stammering experts as the ideas presented in the book are developed with experience and positive feedback from the practitioners.

We will present a different approach.

The Concept of Stammering

Stammering follows a fixed system to trigger speech impediments. A person facing the challenge of stammering is in a state of calm when not speaking. Moments before speaking this person starts to feel anxiety which rises exponentially. The conscious mind will keep looking for the words to be spoken by the person. The presence of difficult words or letters in the sentence to be spoken would raise anxiety even further. This apprehension would be assisted by psychological fear of speaking, which is developed over years of bad experiences. The speaking organs, breathing and the whole body responds to it disturbing the smooth flow of speech. And, the stammering happens. This becomes a self-perpetuating vicious cycle, constantly feeding the subconscious mind about the inability of speaking certain letters or words. This automatic process happens instantly, in a fraction of a second.

To defeat stammering, this automatic system of triggering the anxiety must initially be disturbed, then broken. The subconscious mind needs to be freed from the wrong beliefs about our speech impediments and replaced with the confidence to speak fluently, without stammering.

We will aim to achieve this objective in this book.

Never Stop Practicing

People who have successfully defeated stammering through disciplined and consistent practice have experienced relapses of stammering once they stop practicing. Stammering is a rigid habit that does not leave its victims easily. It sits deep inside the subconscious mind waiting to be activated automatically for some specific letters or words, creating speech impediments. It is triggered automatically in a person who is unaware of the pattern or process of the trigger. They only experience the exponential rise of anxiety, rapidly, due to deep-seated psychological fear of a few letters. We will refer to them as problem letters or difficult letters.

Stammering is a habit that will take disciplined practice to defeat. In most cases, stammering can show signs of weakness without getting weakened. Just like any action story, the protagonist becomes complacent, lowering his guards and allowing the enemy to strike again. Similarly, with sincere practice, the stammering will seem to accept defeat, only to fictitiously convince you of a fake victory. As the practice is stopped to enjoy the newfound freedom to speak without obstructions, stammering attacks again, coming back in full force.

If this behavior of stammering is understood, we cannot be deceived by it. We need to act smart. The solution is simple, never stop practicing. Once we are convinced that stammering is defeated and six months have passed without any signs of strength, practice can slowly be reduced in intensity. It is suggested to keep at least 25% of the intensity always to keep stammering away from your psychological borders. This simply means that you can reduce the intensity of your practice but never stop it completely to sustain your victory over stammering.

The Facts

Let me share some data and information about stammering to have a better understanding of this problem.

About 1% of the human population stammers. This percentage generally remains the same in almost all regions, languages, races and people of a different color. If we include mild cases of stammering then this percentage will rise to 2-3%. The world has around 5-10% of people with speech disorders.

Stammering generally starts as developmental stammering- the stammering which starts during childhood before the age of five. 1 child in 20 stammers before the age of 5 which changes to 1 in 100 by teenage years and adulthood. If we include the mild cases then this number will increase to 3 in 100. Neurological stammering cases are rare, which is either since birth or due to an accident or disease. We will not be covering the solution to these cases in this book.

People with stammering can be intelligent and are capable in every aspect, just the way any other normal person is. There is no link between stammering and intelligence. Stuttering does not affect intelligence in any way.

As a small percentage of people stammer and is not considered life-threatening, just the way color deficiency is, therefore less focus and funds are allotted to it. People with stammering understand its challenge and look for quick solutions in the form of medication or operative procedures and fall to many frauds waiting to exploit their frustration. Therefore, be careful when you look for solutions and do not do anything which seems irrational, fictitious or uncomfortable.

The gender ratio of people with stammering is 1:4 for females and males. It means that males have four times more chances than females to stammer. Also, for every one female who stammers, four males are struggling with the same problem.

Stammering started in early age (before the age of 5) is comparatively less rigid than stammering setting at a later age. Higher the age of stammering (the time a person has lived with stammering), the deeper it sits in the subconscious mind, hence harder it is to defeat. With age and maturity, the fear and anxiety for words become less intense, leading to a slight reduction in stammering, but it becomes more rigid. Most cases of developmental stammering can be corrected to a high percentage (even above 95%) with discipline and perseverance.

In the UK and its past colonies, the habit of speech impediments is called stammering while in all other places of the world it is called stuttering. In this book, we will use both these words interchangeably, which describe the same problem.

We believe that people with stammering are destined to do great things in their lives, as they have suffered enough with their unrealized potential. Only they need to believe it and take action to release their untapped energy.

The Philosophy

What is the fundamental problem? What are our experiences and belief? What is the philosophy of our solution to defeat stammering?

Based on our understanding, research and experience, the fundamental reason for most cases of stammering is the presence of a wrong belief in the subconscious mind. This belief has been built over several years of bad experiences. The subconscious mind cannot be controlled consciously, instead, it is an automatic reaction to some event for which it is conditioned. To defeat stammering, the first step would be to correct these wrong beliefs sitting deep in the subconscious mind, which are responsible for triggering anxiety, leading to stammering. We will aim to correct it.

Is it possible to change a deep-seated belief in the subconscious mind? Yes, it can be achieved with constant practice to repeatedly convince the subconscious mind consciously, about our ability to speak well. Through disciplined practice, we can weaken the wrong belief, which is responsible for the automatic triggering of stammering, and replace it with the correct belief about our ability to speak brilliantly.

The mind can correct itself with hard conscious practice. It can be trained to be disconnected from anxiety in the presence of another person, allowing fluent speaking, with minimal or nil impediments. Always know your limits to prevent excessive physical strain. If you practice enough, the mind will not trigger anxiety and hence stammering. This is one of the aims of the ideas presented in this book.

The Approach to the Problem

Our approach to the problem is simple but effective. This approach has worked wonders for the people with stammering.

To keep everything simple and easy to understand we would use a commonsense-based approach. Exercises and techniques presented would feel intuitive and logical.

We do not believe in medication, psychiatric treatment or operational procedures to cure stammering. It is a habit that requires genuine personal efforts to break free from it.

According to our understanding, stuttering is a rigid habit that triggers anxiety due to psychological fear of few letters or words. The speaking organs of the person who stammers are functioning properly. This claim is correct as a person who stammers can speak normally alone or in certain situations with controlled anxiety, like while singing, when they do not hear their voice or while speaking in front of children.

We believe that the most effective cure is to learn from the people who have cured themselves. We can learn from their ideas, exercises and techniques, which can be modified or customized based on requirements and limitations.

Adamant with Time

Developmental stammering which starts at an early age, around the age of five, is cured easily. Only 1 in 100 carry it to adulthood. Stammering which develops later in life is stubborn and requires dedicated efforts to defeat it. Stammering sits deep in the subconscious mind. It keeps getting deeper with the passing months and years. This means that the longer the time a person has lived with stammering, the higher the resistance he will face to solve it. In the case of stammering, earlier is better. It should be understood that stammering does not attain depth in the subconscious mind in a few months, instead it takes several years to decades to raise solid opposition to your efforts. This does not mean that a person with long-standing stammering cannot solve it, instead, a higher level of commitment and effort would be required to defeat stammering, which becomes part of the person's behavior.

An adult living with stammering for a long time, shifts its priority to lower levels, as other important issues get importance and their attention. Most of their daily energy is consumed by major issues of life and work, leaving nothing to focus on their speech problems. Only in rare and extraordinary situations, does stammering gets its priority back.

In the effort to live with stammering, people get into jobs where speaking well is not required, therefore they do not feel the need for a solution. They create their unique systems to avoid speaking or they speak minimally.

Solving the problem of stammering would require a long time, hard work, commitment and consistency, which could be hard or complex for people to manage. They discover creative reasons to procrastinate.

People who have lived long with stammering accept it as a way of life. They learn to live with it and do not find it uncomfortable. They tend to become immune to mockery and humiliation and people accept them with speech limitations. The intensity of the 'need' to get freedom from stammering loses steam. This disturbs the commitment to defeat stammering, which directly affects their actions against it. For older people who have lived long with stammering, makes it a part of their life. They cannot visualize a life without their rigid stammering, it is their way of speaking.

Do not wait to solve the problem of stammering. Start now.

Efforts Do Fail

As stammering is a rigid habit, defeating it is difficult. It may take consistent long efforts and practice. Many people who have repeatedly failed to defeat stammering tend to lose hope and start to blame themselves. Any new effort to speak without impediments is bound to fail as they do not believe their abilities to defeat stammering. The first and one of the most important elements to defeat stammering is to train the mind for regular practice, with self-belief.

Most adults (with stuttering problems) have lived with stammering for years, even decades. A large percentage of these adults have learned to live with stammering. They do not find it limiting or troubling. This does not allow them to generate the required internal force for hard actions, which is necessary to defeat stammering. This means that most of their efforts would be shallow, never leading to any positive output. These repeated failures reinforce their belief in their inability to get freedom from stammering.

Even though communication is an important part of every human being but people learn to live life with speech impediments. Other priorities replace the need to speak well without difficulties. They get busy in their personal life, work and entertainment, leaving the hope to speak well behind. They start to believe, fallaciously, that stammering is invincible. To defeat stammering it is necessary to have hope and rekindle the excitement of communicating impressively.

The fundamental idea of this book is based on the speaking practice to defeat stammering. Each of the specified exercises and techniques is powerful to develop a person into a good speaker. It is important to choose the right exercises and techniques for regular practice. In many cases, people are unable to choose suitable exercises which do not deliver the required value. Sometimes, the methodology used for practice is not proper, the efforts are not enough, energy is lacking or the direction is not right. But, with constant practice, any practitioner can identify the right and suitable ideas for himself.

People with stammering and their families are generally under mental stress to get the solution. Sometimes, they get trapped with the wrong people promising miracles with the sole objective of extracting money from the victims. These bad experiences are frustrating enough to lose trust in any solution promising the freedom from stammering. These people stop trying, losing any hope to speak better.

The impact of the presented exercises and techniques would multiply with constant feedback and modifications for improvement. Regular feedback of the results from practice must be taken to personalize the exercises and techniques. These changes ensure better impact.

It is important to start the practice to defeat stammering with energy and motivation, as without it results will not be achieved. Many people take the project to defeat stammering without commitment or any intention for sincerity. This means that their efforts remain half-hearted.

Sometimes, people with their bad experiences or the influence of others tend to believe in the permanency of stammering, which means that they can never free themselves from stammering. They will even deny the facts of people who successfully cured stammering to become good speakers. Without the belief in self and in the solution, the desired results will not be achieved.

Sometimes, people in the haste to implement the solution starts the practice without committing to it. This leads to early burnout due to superficial actions. Nothing of importance can be achieved without complete focus, promise and honesty.

As specified before, the struggle to defeat stammering will take time, many months to a few years. If this time duration is not accepted due to an illogical rush to get freedom from stammering, then regularity of practice cannot be maintained. Discipline is necessary to get results. It must be understood that the project is going to be long-term and if it is left midway then the achieved improvements can be reversed.

Sometimes, people get frustrated due to delays in getting the first visible results, which may take a few months to many months. Due to the lack of patience, some people may leave even if they gain confidence in speaking. The aim should be to practice constantly forcing stammering to accept defeat.

Many people who have successfully won over stammering get frustrated due to its relapse. Stammering has the habit of coming back once the practice stops. Some people in excitement to get the command over spoken words, stop practicing the exercises which helped defeat stammering. This mistake may lead to frustration as stammering regains control over our speech. A small percentage of people accept stammering the part of their life as they lose motivation to start again.

To keep stammering/ stuttering away would require constant efforts and consistent practice. Any failure to keep regularity and discipline would bring stuttering back.

What is Stammering

Stammering is present with humanity since the time languages were developed and humans started to interact. The main reasons for the development of the habit of stammering remain the same, anxiety and lack of confidence. As ancient people did not have the privilege of a structured language and a large part of the communication was through body language, the impact of stammering was limited. But, as the language developed and social structure became organized the level of anxiety in communication kept increasing. This can be considered the beginning of stammering for the human species. Even the people speaking normally tend to stammer during the state of anxiety or fear. Stammering is worse, as the trigger to a specific word sits deep in the subconscious mind waiting to activate the resistance to speaking. This would lead to stammering.

Before moving forward let's understand the concept of stammering. What is stammering and what is not? In many cases, the loss of words or inability to pronounce certain words does not imply that the person stammers. In other cases, due to some neurological problems stammering can occur which is due to the lack of proper connection between the mind and speech. For example, in certain cases after stroke (generally due to high blood pressure in older people) patients may tend to stammer while speaking. Other people may have speaking defects since birth which may also be connected to some neurological disorders. We need to understand that these cases are not due to psychological fear of words, instead, they are neurological disorders that would require an expert or doctor for diagnosis and treatment through medication or surgical procedures.

In this book, we have covered only the aspect of developmental disorders or the problems which are generally due to the psychological fear of certain letters or words. In these cases, the person who stammers can speak properly when alone but would have difficulty in speaking the same phrases or words in front of an audience or other people, which is generally due to anxiety, restlessness and fear of words. This book is focused on the techniques to deal with anxiety and fear which are the major impediments to communicating properly.

Stammering is when:

• you repeat sounds or syllables – for example, such as saying "mu-mu-mu-mummy"

• you make sounds longer – for example, "mmmmmmummy"

• a word gets stuck or doesn't come out at all

a person who stammers is distinctly visible when he struggles to speak certain words to express himself. Some people may consider the anxiety, hesitation and the struggle of the person who stammers as comical or hilarious but they are unable to understand the frustration, the pain and the weight of fear which doubles when that person is unable to communicate properly. The irresponsible actions of other people also become the cause of enhancing the fear of words for the person who was already struggling with words.

Stammering varies in severity from person to person, and from situation to situation. Someone might have periods of stammering followed by times when they speak relatively fluently.

Some people may call stammering a disease. It can even be categorized as a disease, which many do, but it delivers a negative message to the sufferer and their family members. These words unnecessarily amplify the anxiety and fear levels of these people. If we call stammering a habit or a hard-ingrained behavior then it implies that the habit can be changed or the behavior can be improved. This book will call stammering a habit that can be cured through hard practice and the right techniques.

Stammering also has the habit of relapsing, if it is taken lightly. The techniques and practices responsible for defeating stammering must not be loosened, as speech impediments may bounce back. It implies to keep practicing, even if with lower intensity, the chosen techniques, methodology and ideas which have led to improvement in your speech and communication.

Types of Stammering

About 1% (2-3% including mild cases) of the people in the world stammer. The reasons for stammering could be:

1. **Developmental stammering**: These cases are mainly due to stammering starting during the developmental phase, which is early childhood (around age 3-5), when the speech was being developed. This stammering is mainly due to the lack of words or the grammar rules or the clarity of thinking. Around 5% of the kids face developmental stammering and out of which 80% are cured naturally, while the remaining one-fifth of children carry the problem of stammering to their adulthood.
2. **Late childhood and teenage stammering**: In other cases, stammering can be developed in the childhood or teenage phase when they experience humiliation or mockery due to their inability to speak some words. This develops psychological fear of the specific letter or words in their subconscious mind. This fear strengthens and deepens its roots with passing time, building into the habit of stammering.
3. **Momentary stammering**: This type of stammering is due to momentary anxiety or restlessness. This type of stammering can happen to anyone and the solution lies in dealing with the problem of anxiety. This type of stammering can also be due to uncontrolled breathing patterns.
4. **Speaking fast problem**: Some people develop the habit of speaking extremely fast which they are unable to manage. Due to the speed of speech, they are unable to speak coherently and with control. This is a habit that they could have developed early in their life. For them, this problem was unrecognized and left unattended,

which later developed into a full-fledged problem.

5. **Neurological stammering**: This type of stammering is due to certain connection problems between the mind and speaking organs of a person. Some children have this problem by birth. Adults may develop it during accidents or surgical operations. We will not be covering neurological stammering in this book and it would require diagnosis and treatment by a doctor or medical professional.

Myths of Stammering

There are many myths and wrong beliefs associated with stammering, let's bust them.

- People think that it is a permanent handicap or that stammerers are not normal. Stammering is a habit that develops in childhood and becomes stiff with time. Stammering can be defeated with disciplined efforts.
- Developmental stammering is not a permanent damage in the brain, it is only the psychological fear which is sitting deep in the subconscious mind, triggering anxiety. Only the cases of neurological stammering which are either due to a disease, accident or by birth, would require medical attention.
- The intelligence, logical thinking and creativity of stammerers are in no way less than the people who speak normally without speech impediments.
- People may think that stammering cannot be cured as they have seen elders struggling with stammering. The habit of stammering can be defeated with regular and disciplined practice. Many people have won over

stammering to achieve success in life.

- Some people are deceived to take heavy medication to cure 'the disease of stammering'. Some are even fooled to accept operating procedures. Stammering does not require any medication of any type or any operational procedures to cure it. It is a habit that requires similar actions to break any other habit.
- There is no need for the readjustment of the voice box to cure stammering. The speaking organs of the people with stammering are fine and healthy, they don't need any correction or treatment. Anyone in doubt can check that stammerers speak fluently when alone.
- Stammering is not a curse due to your present or past life deeds. It is absurd to accept this reasoning.
- "You are lazy". People with stammering are not lazy, they are trying extra hard to speak normally. They must have taken several actions to speak normally but they could have failed. To speak normally without impediments remains the greatest desire of every stammerer and they are ready to toil for it.

Initial Points to Keep in Mind

It is important to understand a few points before starting your journey. This path will take you towards a more confident, better speaking person and a strong personality. It will require discipline and commitment to follow through, till stammering is defeated.

Only in a few cases, the problems of stammering are solved in months, instead of years. For most, it is a long struggle for years before they transform themselves into a confident speaker. Consider it a long-term project which should not be paused or stopped till you achieve the desired results.

Consistency will be the key to winning over stammering. Just like in any physical exercise, results cannot be achieved without regularity. Constant efforts with discipline will form the backbone of the whole effort.

You must remember that stammering thrives on strong emotions, therefore you must learn to control them. Panic, anger, frustration, excitement, anxiety, impatience and indiscipline would be your biggest enemies. This is true not only in the present project but in every other task or work.

To defeat stammering we must weaken it and improve our communication skills. Our main objective will be to strengthen our various elements of communication using different exercises and techniques. Simultaneously, we will learn to control our fears and manage anxiety, which will directly improve our speaking by minimizing speech impediments.

As we are presenting a large number of exercises and techniques, it is important to check and test each one of them to select the most suitable exercises and techniques. In your daily practice, you must be aware of the results you are achieving through regular feedback. You can modify these ideas to have a better impact based on your unique environment and conditions. If anything is not working for you then leave it and adopt anything else which is working towards solving the problem.

Stammering has the habit of relapsing or coming back. It has been observed that the people who had successfully defeated their stammering but stopped practicing the exercises, experienced stammering raising its head again. This means that we must continue practicing even after we become confident speakers. We can come out of the practice schedule slowly but systematically.

In the end, you will realize that stammering was a blessing in disguise. It allowed you to focus on developing your personality and communication skills. Most people aren't enough motivated for this level of commitment and focus. The competencies developed in the process of defeating stammering help a person in career and various aspects of personal life. This truth has been proven by the high achievements of the people with stammering.

In this book, we will deal only with developmental stammering, which generally develops during childhood and persists in adulthood. In this discussion, we will not cover neurological stammering, which is either by birth, due to an accident or started after a disease. For these cases, please take suggestions from medical doctors and specialists.

The initial results may not be visible immediately even after a few weeks of constant efforts. Do not stop practicing and training to defeat your stammering. In some cases, the initial results will be visible after a few weeks, for others it may take a few months, while some cases may take a couple of years. Your constant practice would surely weaken and finally defeat your stammering, stuttering or speech impediments.

CHAPTER TWO

Mental Training

> *"Winning is something that builds physically and mentally every day that you train and every night that you dream."*

Emmitt Smith

It is all in Mind

Your journey to defeat stammering will require sincerity, commitment and discipline. This project can be long, taking years of regular practice. In some cases, it may even relapse, resetting your progress to make you push forward again. It may constitute many other challenges in your professional and personal lives. This process would require a certain time commitment, every day, to practice exercises. Many other challenges, based on your unique conditions and environment may raise their heads to slow your progress. To win over stammering a resilient head and strong willpower would be required.

Mental training is also necessary to get maximum value from the exercises and techniques presented in the book. Consistent efforts would be required to improve your speaking, as without regularity the required force to defeat stammering will not be generated. This segment will also discuss the main points that you must always keep in mind while working on your speaking skills. Just like any other exercise starts with a warm-up, mental training would be the warm-up to start your drills. Before starting with any of the exercises or techniques you must be mentally ready to enjoy it and use it to its maximum effects. In addition to these ideas to train your mind, you can also introspect based upon the points discussed in the book, to extract maximum value from ideas.

Mental training is an important section of the whole process to improve speaking skills. It should not be ignored or avoided. You may need to give a few days or a week to train your mind for effectively starting your practice. Once the mind is ready to defeat stammering, you will surely be a winner.

Truth Acceptance

The first and an important aspect of mental training is to accept the truth that the problem of stammering exists. Many people try to ignore this fact, trying to fabricate illogical reasons for it. This attitude adds to their pre-existing fear. The anxiety multiplies, deteriorating the problem of stammering. This is to be understood that ignoring the facts will never solve the problem. It must be taken head-on. To start, introspect the problem in speaking and assess the work required to solve it. Take a few days or even a week to get clarity in mind before starting the project to defeat stammering.

Once the truth is accepted, the following changes can be experienced:

- The feeling of self-confidence for crossing the mental barrier of speaking the truth to yourself. This is a moment of pride.
- As the first step has been taken the stress will slowly start to loosen its grip.
- Once the truth is accepted, a part of the fear is already defeated.
- This is proof of the existence of not only the desire but also the readiness to take action to defeat stammering.
- The willpower is activated to take on the challenges that lie ahead.
- A fraction of your stammering is already defeated.

The Belief

People who aren't able to solve their problem of stammering have accepted it as a part of their life, a part of their body. That is the reason they never get mentally ready to eradicate stammering to become a better speaker. This wrong thinking gives rise to the belief that stammering is permanent and they can never defeat it. Once this idea sets in mind, stammering becomes the winner as that individual is not ready to challenge it. This must change.

To defeat stammering and become a better speaker you must believe that it can be defeated and you possess the right abilities to defeat it. This is the next step after accepting the problem of stammering. You must stop complaining or whining about the impediments in your speech, instead commit to take on the hard steps to win over your stammering.

To start believing in yourself and your abilities again, you must keep repeating these facts in your mind and take hard steps towards initial successes. This is possible through rational actions. Once you taste initial success, the mind will start to believe in your abilities to speak impressively.

Commitment and Regularity

Every day many people think about many goals, big goals, but only a fraction of people take action towards them and few achieve it. That is a simple difference between the people who get results and the people who give reasons. The only difference between these two segments of people is their commitment to achieve results. This promise generates the required force to push you forward towards your goals and make you achieve your targets. This is something of utmost importance to defeat stammering. The commitment will drive you forward, even in hard times, to keep moving towards the desired goals. So, commit now to defeat your stammering.

We know about the importance of regularity to build your muscles with physical exercises. Similar conformity is required to learn a new subject or to develop something. The efforts to defeat stammering will be effective only if they are regular, consistent and without gaps.

So, before starting your efforts to defeat stammering, commit to being regular in your endeavors.

Sincerity with Discipline

Once you commit to something, it would require complete sincerity to achieve your goals. It means that you are completely honest about your efforts and are ready to put in the required work. This is necessary as most people diminish their intensity of practice, without considering that it may lead to their defeat instead of stammering. We also need to understand that our actions are not a showcase for anybody else, but ourselves.

Sincerity goes hand in hand with discipline. The best example is the military or a school, where discipline forms the backbone of the whole system. It leads to results. This concept is also true for every organization, institution or company. Each has a set of rules, both specified or unspecified, which have to be strictly followed for the organization to achieve its objectives. Discipline is also necessary for any project or task which is required to be completed within deadlines and with the required quality.

A disciplined schedule must be designed for your practice to defeat stammering, which must be sincerely followed without breaks or gaps. If any break in practice happens then redesign your schedule and start again. Keep repeating this process till you get the command over your spoken words.

Patience- It will Take Time

The world has changed drastically from the generations of the last century. Powerful devices, high-speed Internet and featured apps have allowed split second messages, content sharing and multi-player gaming. Online stores allow you to buy anything of unending varieties, instantly. These facilities have changed the beliefs and expectations of normal human beings. They want everything without delay or wait. But this will not be the case in the fight to defeat stammering.

Stammering is a rigid habit that sits deep in the subconscious mind of a person. It has gained strength over the years since childhood. It can only be defeated by consistent disciplined practice to defeat this habit. It cannot be done instantly. A person who believes in himself/herself must be ready to put in years of hard work to win the right to speak confidently, fluently and without fear.

Patience would be the requirement in your journey to have command over your spoken words. This path will be hard but, in the end, you will be a transformed person, not only in speaking but also in various other attributes of personality. Once your mind accepts this reality, it will automatically help you in your struggle against stammering with patience.

Do not take this journey as a punishment, instead consider this time for self-improvement and self-discovery. Make it fun.

Let Go of the Hesitation and Fear

Every person who stammers has experienced mockery of some kind from others. Some people make fun of them and laugh demeaningly at the cost of their self-esteem. You must understand that only a few people will sympathize with your suffering. You should not expect any sympathy from anyone, as the expectation of compassion would make your confidence contingent on their actions. You must be self-sufficient to deal with your problems on your own, without support from anyone. That is the level of mental toughness required in your battle against stammering. You should not be affected by the reactions of other people to remain focused on your goals.

To start, you must free yourself from the threads of hesitation, and develop an attitude of a participant. You must take part in all the public speaking evens like debates, presentations, speeches, theater and speaking up your mind in the class or meetings. You may stammer on stage, triggering a weird reaction from the listeners, but that should not discourage you from speaking. You should not miss any chance to speak publicly, share your opinion, give information and persuade people about your ideas.

The more you follow this suggestion the less anxiety you will feel about speaking and the reactions of other people. This will directly affect your speaking by reducing anxiety and stress levels. As stammering is connected to anxiety, you will observe lesser instances of speech impediments.

From this moment onwards you must commit not to hesitate about using spoken words, whenever you feel the need to speak. Whatever happens, you must cross every hurdle to make speaking one of your strengths.

Touch the Limits of Practice

Several times people have doubts that since everybody is working hard in their job, why only a few are gliding towards more responsibility and better profiles, while others are struggling to survive in their existing jobs. The reason is hidden in the performance, which can be identified by the quality of results achieved, and the untapped hidden potential of the person. The professionals who are considered "doers", people who get things done, are loved and nurtured by every organization. These are the people who put their best into the task given to them while enjoying the whole process. They keep learning with the desire to keep growing constantly. They learn new skills and develop new competencies. Management admires them and their colleagues desire to emulate them. Their secret is hidden in the discipline and the sincerity towards their work. They never take their job casually, instead, follow the principle of kaizen, which is growing and improving every day. They are never satisfied with their high-performance levels as they believe that a lot more is yet to be achieved. They believe in their abilities to touch their limits and push them further. This is exactly what you must do to defeat stammering.

You must remember that your consistent and disciplined efforts would defeat stammering. Your success in improving your speaking abilities will depend on your hard practice. You should try to touch your limits, without hurting yourself in any way, and then push them further. This will ensure that your level of training will keep improving to weaken stammering.

The optimum level for each exercise and technique has been specified, but if you can do more then do it. The more you practice the faster you will gain control over your spoken words. Define the schedule for yourself and keep improving it with experience.

Never be causal about your training with exercises, techniques and with other methods.

Time Factor

Most people who are unable to solve the problem of stammering tried to solve it, but they didn't try long enough. These people followed the right process, they worked hard with discipline and regularity, but they lacked the patience to follow through. They stopped early, as they hoped for prompt results. Stammering is a rigid habit that takes constant efforts for a certain time to weaken its grip on the person. It can vary from a few months to even more than a year. People who were waiting for immediate results will lack the patience to keep working without testing initial successes. Even though we have discussed many ideas to get results within a few weeks of effort, defeating it completely will require a long time. Those unable to accept this fact will have a lower probability to win over stammering.

Even before starting your first exercise or technique, you must accept the fact that this project will require work commitment for years. A few cases may see a drastic improvement in a few months of practice, but for most cases, it will be more than a year or more. Once this fact is accepted, your practice will become part of your daily routine. The regularity of training will be the key differentiating factor. Even if you do not see desired results in initial few months, you should not loosen your efforts.

Keep working fervently and believe in yourself. You will surprise yourself with your performance and results.

Understand that it may Relapse

Stammering sits deep in the subconscious mind triggering anxiety and fear for words and letters. Years of hard practice is required to defeat it. Stammering is rigid and does not accept defeat easily. It may show signs of weakness after regular training, but it may return. In many cases, stammering may seem to subside by 80%-90%, but as the person loosens his daily practice, it storms back. Be aware of this fact. It means that even if the command over spoken words is achieved, the efforts to achieve it should not be reduced. Regular speaking training can be slowly reduced in intensity in phases only after six months of uninterrupted fine speaking. Around 200 days of confident speaking is enough time to convince the subconscious mind about our speaking abilities. After completing the specified period, the intensity of exercises can be slowly reduced. But, never stop your practice completely. Finally, keep at least fifteen minutes of regular speaking practice to prevent stammering gaining strength again.

Remember to keep your practice regularly at least for a few minutes every day to keep stammering away and to keep improving your communication skills. Never stop practicing.

CHAPTER THREE

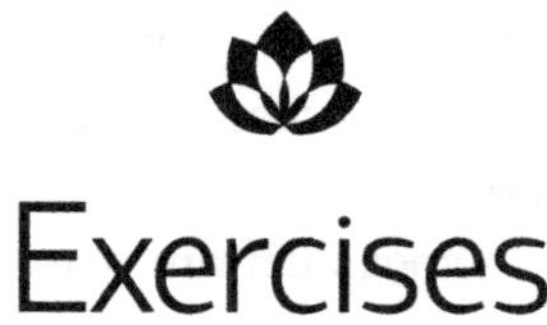

Exercises

Defeat Hesitation in Speaking

Fear of speaking gives birth to the hesitation of speaking and this hesitation is responsible for amplifying stammering. Hesitation is having severe self-doubts forcing you to develop a reluctance to act. This habit then falls into the vicious loop, in which more hesitation develops more fear which aggravates the habit of hesitation. The confidence goes down, self-doubts appear and people hide themselves inside self-created shells. They spend a long time inside their mental and physical shells. During this time their stammering gains rigidity, becoming stubborn. This impasse can be broken if we decide not to hesitate. The moment you complete reading this topic you must decide to kill hesitation forever. You must not hesitate in speaking anywhere even if you have difficulty delivering a smooth flow of spoken words. If you are asked to give a presentation you must present, if someone requests you for the speech you must come forward and even if no one is asking you to speak even then you must find the opportunity to walk towards the stage. You can find a large number of opportunities to speak like debates, extempore, discussions, QA, sharing your opinion and reciting poems. Once you become immune to others' reactions toward you, your speaking skills would instantly become better.

In short, you must not leave any opportunity to speak. You may have hesitation or fear of speaking, but you must ignore it. It is also possible that the worst happens on stage and you are unable to speak certain words or you stammer, but persevere. Once you decide to speak then slowly the hesitation will fade away. You must accept that people will behave the way they have always behaved, you cannot change them. You should not try to change anybody for their ill behavior. But, you can change yourself immediately by throwing out your hesitation in speaking. Start doing it from this moment onwards.

Book Reading

Every day we consume a lot of information in the form of text, audio or video. We read newspapers, watch television and listen to audiobooks. This technique simply stresses the importance of reading text aloud, whenever possible. This does not mean to disturb anybody with your voice in the library, at school or during a meeting, instead use this idea to practice speaking.

Stammering can be defeated with regular speaking practice, we must find the opportunities to speak with clear words. Reading the text aloud can be one way to practice speaking in the best possible way. For example, if you are reading a novel, it can be read aloud just the way you can read a news article or a nonfiction book.

The best place to read aloud can be the personal space of your home, office cabin or car. You must ensure that every word coming out of your mouth must be crystal clear, it must not be spoken casually. Never drag during reading, your reading must be effective enough to impress an audience.

Start using this simple technique from the next possible moment onwards. In the coming weeks and months, you will notice improved control over spoken words. With regular practice, speaking fluently will become normal for you and a part of your habit.

Precautions:

- Use this technique rationally without disturbing others in any way or attracting the unwanted attention of others.
- Use it reasonably to extract the required value from this technique.

Tongue Twisters

Communication is the backbone of human development. It is responsible for thinking, generation of ideas, development of innovative solutions and sharing them with others for improvisation and enhancement. Communication also defines the success of an organization, institution, individual and even nations. The way we think and communicate our feelings to others is one of the best discovery by humanity. Without language, homo sapiens had no chance in ruling planet earth. For effective thinking, clarity of ideas is important. Without an organized thought process, we would be lost in a twisted mess of noise in mind. This undesirable confusion can never lead to anything productive. Once we have clarity of thought in our mind, then only it can be transferred to others. Ideas, feelings and human thought are communicated through spoken words. The power of words delivered from the mouth can influence the hearts and minds of people. Politician, corporate brands and celebrities use them effectively. The communication language used must be simple with clarity of message delivered. For oral communication, quality of word pronunciation is as important as the ideas it contains. A small percentage of people have clear pronunciation in oral communication. Everyone knows about its importance, but are unable to put required efforts to improve their pronunciation in their spoken language.

Most people also lack the required tools and techniques to bring clarity in their speech.

Quality in words pronunciation is appreciated by all, irrespective of the spoken language. That is necessary for fine and effective speech, which is required in all professional and personal endeavors. Many capable people fail to achieve their potential due to lack of good communication skills. An effective way to deliver the ideas and messages is a must for personal and professional success. This fact had always been correct, it is true now and it will remain valid in the distant future.

According to Oxford dictionary a 'Tongue Twister' is "a sequence of words or sounds, typically of an alliterative kind, that is difficult to pronounce quickly and correctly, as, for example, 'tie twine to three tree twigs'. Tongue Twisters are the combination of words to form a phrase or sentence which are difficult to speak repeatedly while speaking at normal or fast speed. Practicing with Tongue Twisters is a good exercise to improve pronunciation and control over spoken words. Each tongue twister can focus on a specific letter or a combination of letters. Alliteration is used to create rhetorical impact through repetition of same sounds or the same kinds of sounds at the start of the words or in the stressed syllables, beginning either with a consonant or a vowel, in close succession. This can be used in clauses, phrases or sentences. The phrases (alliterations and/or tongue twisters) can be used to bring clarity in their pronunciation and speech through regular intensive practice.

To practice, Tongue Twisters must be spoken aloud repeatedly, at least seven times. We suggest repeating each of the phrases ten times, consistently without pause, with their above average spoken speed. The most important part is fluency and the clarity in pronunciation for each spoken word. You can record your practice sessions to check for the pronunciation clarity of words. Start the speaking practice of tongue twisters with slow speed and gradually increase your phrase delivery speed to your maximum limit. These exercises would be straining on the lungs, tongue, neck, and mouth. Every person has different capacity, so know your limits and care must be taken to avoid injury of any form. With constant practice, the readers would notice a gradual improvement in clarity of speech, word pronunciation and command on spoken words. Readers can use these phrases in their unique, innovative or personalized ways to speak and practice (for their speech clarity).

Breathing Exercises 1234

Breathing is one of the most important elements for speaking properly and impressively. It is surprising to note that most people are not using this powerful and natural way to make themselves healthy and have better control over their lives. Our breaths have become shallow and nonrhythmic. The reasons could be pollution, lifestyle, stress or sleep deprivation. In a few cases, the lack of control over breathing impacts our speaking negatively. Inability to breathe naturally affects our ability to speak smoothly. A stammering person would experience anxiety and irregular breathing, which will impede his speech. To defeat stammering we must have complete control over our breathing.

This exercise has the following objectives:

- To have control over our breathing,
- To have natural rhythmic breathing,
- To have deep breathing to reduce anxiety, and
- To relax and reduce stress.

How to do it:

- Sit in a comfortable position in a quiet place, where you will not be disturbed for some time.
- We will do this exercise by closing our eyes as it requires complete focus.
- Every breath, both inhaled or exhaled, must be deep.
- We will breathe in from the nose and breathe out from the mouth.
- We will count one, two, three, four with the time duration of one second in each count for every breathing activity.

- The complete breathing exercise would involve three activities, that is breathing in, pausing and breathing out.
- We will breathe in by counting from 1 to 4 in our minds with the difference of one second between each number. We will hold our breath by counting 1 to 4 in our minds for the difference of one second between each number. The last activity of this exercise would be to breathe out by counting from 1 to 4 in our minds with the difference of one second between each number. In short, we will start by inhaling in four seconds, then pausing for four seconds and finally exhaling in four seconds. This is one set. We will keep repeating this set, as per our requirements.
- While we are breathing in, we can visualize that cool and pure air filling our brain and our lungs with freshness. While we are holding our breath for four seconds, we can visualize that all our stress, anxiety and muscle strain are getting sucked out of our body. In the final step, while breathing out, we can visualize that all the stress, anxiety, strain, fear and pain are going out of our body through our mouth, in the form of hot exhaled air. We are now left with mental peace and calmness.
- You can do this exercise 4 times a day with 10 repetitions.

Precautions:

- If you have any breathing problems (like asthma) then you will need to consult your doctor before doing this exercise.

- If you are not comfortable with the exercise then you should discontinue it and choose any other exercise.

Pen Exercises

Pen Exercises are performed with the help of a pen, pencil or any other similar objects which are safe to hold in your mouth. The objective of this exercise is to create an obstruction using a pen to block the movement of the tongue, lips and jaw. We will speak while holding the pen in our mouth in a certain way. It will be difficult to speak without clarity in the spoken words. Same words, phrases or sentences, if spoken after removing the pen, would allow you to have more control over those words. You will now speak them better than normal. Regular practice of this exercise would allow you to have more control and confidence over your spoken words. In addition to using normal text, use words and sentences containing letters that create difficulties in your speech.

We will use four different ways to hold the pen with our mouth, two with teeth and the other two with lips.

Holding pen with teeth:

Exercise 1

Hold the pen the way a cigarette is held with teeth. This would make the pen sit lengthwise inside the mouth. Do not push it deep, only around an inch inside or the way you feel comfortable. Now speak the chosen sentences while keeping the pen in position. Do not let your lips or tongue get injured in any way. Keep speaking for 30- 45 seconds more. Now, remove the pen and speak the same sentences, you will experience better control. Repeat this exercise five times more with different sentences of various speaking difficulties.

This exercise will be repeated with three other ways of holding a pen with your mouth.

Exercise 2

In this exercise, teeth will hold the pen across the mouth. This time the position of the pen will be 90 degrees from the previous position. The pen will be held by the middle teeth (prominently visible) and would be behind the front teeth. After holding the pen in this way, the previous exercise would be repeated.

Exercise 3

We will repeat the above exercises now with the help of our lips instead of teeth. For this exercise, the lips would be rolled over the front teeth, so that they are not visible. Hold the pen in the same way as exercise 1, and repeat the whole exercise.

Exercise 4

This is the repetition of exercise 2 while rolling the lips in the same way as exercise 3, over the front teeth.

Other points related to the exercise

- The duration of these exercises would vary from person to person depending upon the stamina of doing each of these exercises. Generally, each of these exercises should be repeated five times every day.

- To make the exercise tougher we can use a thicker pen or pencil for putting bigger obstructions in our speech.
- We can also use a recording device to record the audio of the voice for future listening and analysis.

Precautions:

- Use plastic, wooden pen or pencil which are safe to hold in your mouth. Care must be taken to avoid swallowing anything harmful like paint, ink or pen part.
- Do not use anything metallic as it may harm your lips or teeth.
- The pen or pencil must be clean enough to hold in your mouth.
- Do not push the pen deep inside your mouth. Keep it only around an inch inside.
- Always protect your tongue, lips or other muscle or skin from any type of injury from your teeth or external objects.
- Do not let your cheeks, lips or tongue get too tired.

Obstruction Exercises

Obstruction exercises are the advanced version of the pen exercises. These exercises can be understood with an analogy of running very fast for some time and then drastically reducing our running speed, which will allow us to have more control over our body and speed. Similar is the idea of obstruction exercises. In these exercises, we will obstruct our normal speech and then we will remove that obstruction to find that we can speak those words in a much more controlled and smoother way.

We will try different types of obstructions exercises to create obstructions in our speech and then we will remove those obstructions to speak normally in an improved way.

Exercise 1

In this exercise we will use some thicker cylindrical objects (safe) like carrot, radish, and cucumber which can be utilized to repeat four Pen Exercises. Having a thicker object in the mouth will enhance the intensity of the exercise by creating even bigger obstacles in speaking. Follow the instructions above and also check the precautions.

Exercise 2

In this exercise we will obstruct by filling our mouth with some eatables like pieces of apple or grapes. We must have experienced difficulty in speaking when we have something in our mouth. Speak these sentences again after eating the pieces of fruit in your mouth. You will experience more control and clarity over your words. Regular repetition of these exercises is important.

Exercise 3

If you open your mouth and use your thumbs and fingers to push your cheeks inside. This action will reduce the space in your mouth and would restrict the movement of the tongue and your jaw, obstructing your speech. Repeat the part of the above exercise of speaking some complex sentences or paragraphs in this position. Speak these words again after removing your hand, you will find much more control over your words and speech once the obstruction is removed.

Precaution: Be careful not to push your cheeks too hard to prevent any injury.

Exercise 4

Holding lips together- This is the similar exercise as above but with different speaking obstruction, which will be created by holding the lips together, not allowing them to move. It is as if the lips are zipped together and the mouth cannot be opened. Try speaking in this position and you will feel the obstruction in speaking. Speak again after removing the obstruction and you will have more control over your words.

Exercise 5

Holding jaw down- When we speak our upper jaw is fixed while the lower jaw moves to work in synchronization with the tongue to help us produce the required sounds. If you open your mouth wide and hold your jaw in the lower position then it will create an obstruction to speak. Repeat the speaking exercise as in above.

Exercise 6

Jaws bound together- This exercise the related to the previous exercise with a slight variation. In this exercise, we will keep our jaws together, which means our upper and lower jaw teeth are touching each other. In this position, the space available in our mouth drastically reduces, restricting the movement of the tongue. This position creates an obstruction in the mouth hence above speaking exercise can be repeated.

Talking with the Singing Voice

You must have noticed that when you are singing, stammering is not present. The words, phrases and sentences which create difficulty in speaking, if spoken in the singing voice can easily be uttered, without any obstructions or problems. You can have a similar experience while reciting a poem.

Why does this happen? The normal pattern of speaking is not smooth, instead, it can have sharp corners, just like in a square or rectangle. Words can get stuck in the corners. While singing and to some extent poem recitation has rhythmic words, making the whole utterance smooth. It can be compared with a smooth curvy or wavy flow. Words glide over the curves, so the stammering can be avoided.

The wavy flow of words can be utilized in our daily communication. Though it may seem slightly different from the normal way of speaking, but if used properly it can be used in impressive ways. For example, some of the top speeches of the world have a curvy flow of words. Listen to the speech 'I have a Dream' by Martin Luther King Jr. or some of the top speeches of US Presidents.

How to do it?

You can use the technique of speaking in a singing voice in any sentence or paragraph, at any time of the day. You can check the intensity of the curviness of the spoken words. Keep it to the minimum required. The more you practice, the better you would become at using the technique in normal communication, without sounding odd. Regular practice would also train the subconscious mind about your command and fluency over the language, building confidence to defeat your stammering.

Speaking in Noise

Our conscious mind is the main player responsible for generating anxiety and triggering stammering. As the problem (stammering) letter or words approaches us, our pulse shoots up, breathing becomes inconsistent and the effect of anxiety is felt in the whole body, ensuring stammering on that specific letter. The interpretation of the conscious mind reinforces the belief in the subconscious mind about our stammering. This pattern keeps repeating and so does our stammering. We must weaken this belief in our subconscious mind about our stammering.

One of the training is by convincing the subconscious mind that we can speak normally. This will materialize by proving to the subconscious mind that we can speak normally. You must have observed that when you do not listen to your voice, you do not stammer. This exercise is one of many exercises which will help in proving our ability to speak normally.

When we are present in a controlled noise, a big part of the conscious mind is busy dealing with the content of the noise, segregating the relevant messages from the noise. Also, the noise would restrict the flow of our voice to our ears. This means that we will be able to listen to our voice, but it will be minimal. You must have observed that during attending an Indian marriage, a political rally, a loud market or a rock show would limit the intensity of our voice. That is the time when a stammerer would speak normally or with minimal stammering. If you are unable to listen to your voice then your mind will be unable to make you stutter.

The noise in this exercise would be created in a controlled way. It should not be too loud that hurts the ears in any way, too low will not work. We can use headphones or earphones to listen to a song, a conversation, a speech or even music. The volume of the audio should be loud enough to minimize the flow of your voice to your ears. Now, try to speak something, especially the words containing the difficult letters. You should record your spoken words using another device. Once this exercise is over, you can listen back to the audio to surprise yourself with the normalcy of your speech.

Repeat this exercise for five minutes, 3 to 4 times a week.

Points related to exercise:

- Noise can be in any form. It could be audio from a TV, radio, mobile or it could be a natural sound from the sea (beach), waterfall, river or rainfall. It can even include people talking.
- This exercise involves speaking loud but not shouting, which can be hurtful to your throat. Speaking loud means uttering words that are clear and the speaker has control over the spoken language.

- This would be a different feeling as we have the habit of listening to our voices.
- This exercise would build speaking confidence.
- This exercise is also helpful in building the strength of voice.
- Do this exercise rationally, as speaking loudly is stressful to the throat.

Make Speaking Difficult Exercises

If you are asked to run fast, as fast as possible, it would be extremely straining for your body. But, after a few minutes if you are asked to run comfortably then that would seem extremely easy. The same is the case for problem-solving. To solve a problem, the best way to make any problem simple is by solving harder problems. Your experience with the harder problems would make any other problem relatively simpler.

This is the fundamental philosophy of some of our exercises. We create conditions in which speaking becomes difficult and we practice speaking in those conditions (definitely, in a safe way). Once, we have practiced enough and become comfortable speaking in those conditions, then speaking normally becomes easy. That is one of the keys to defeat the problem of stammering, as previously dominant speech impediments would weaken. Even the normal speakers who want to improve their speaking skills can use these exercises for regular training.

In this book, we have presented some of these exercises. Now, we suggest the learners develop their own innovative exercises using their creative muscles, based on their unique environments and availability of resources. Test these exercises for their effectiveness and keep improving them through feedback.

How to use feedback? Practice the exercise and check the results after 3 to 4 weeks. If you feel that results are as expected then the exercise is working, if not, then make the required modifications or corrections to the exercise and repeat the cycle. This whole process can be called as the 'one iteration of the Feedback Loop'. Keep working on these iterations till expected results are achieved.

Add the final personalized exercises to your list for regular practice. You would be more connected to these exercises as they were enhanced created by your efforts.

In your practice and search for exercises, make sure to keep yourself safe and injury-free.

Visualize and Speak

Visualization is one of the most authoritative tools in creative thinking. Einstein used the power of visualization to discover many laws of physics and stated that "visualization is more powerful than knowledge". His views are shared by innovators and thinkers. Visualization is not restricted to arts, it has a big role in every other field, including science, engineering and technology. Science fiction inspires scientists to work on new technologies and to create high-tech products. Visualization also allows us to ask powerful questions which form the basis for innovation. Entrepreneurs visualize ideas before starting their companies, transforming them into world leaders.

Visualization allows people to look beyond the limitations created by society and the environment in which they live and work. It is heavy on mental resources as it requires complete focus, concentration and deep thinking. Visualization creates a world of its own in mind, that is the reason it can be helpful in our fight against stammering. You need to talk aloud about the world created in your mind while visualizing it.

You can visualize with open eyes too but most fails to reach this level. Powerful visualization is deeply engrossing, capturing the complete attention of the person. This experience is equivalent to meditation as the conscious mind gets busy visualizing and absorbing all details. With regular practice, you learn to get depth in visualization. As the conscious mind is busy with the process of visualization the subconscious mind does not get activated for raising the anxiety level for certain difficult letters, hence the instances of stammering reduce considerably.

How to do it?

- Sit in a comfortable position, where you will not be disturbed.
- This exercise is about visualizing something interesting and speaking it aloud.
- Keep everything normal, including your breathing, and close your eyes to either visit a place, event or create something with your mind like a beautiful park with flowers.
- Now describe the details of each and everything you see. For example, you can talk about the details of the tree which you are watching or the color of the leaves and their unique shape.
- You can go deeper into the details and can even experience your visualization through the senses like

smell, taste, sound and even touch. The more the senses are used the better the experience would become.

- You can do this exercise as long as you want, and as many times as you want.
- This is a type of meditation that will reduce your stress by calming your mind.

Precautions:

- Do not do this exercise when you are walking, driving or doing any physical work, as you can injure yourself.
- Do not speak loud to avoid disturbing others.

Light in Mind

Light in mind is an extremely effective concept that we all know about and have experienced. To understand this concept we need to start from the beginning. When a child is born her mind is completely blank as if it is full of darkness. She cannot understand the language we are speaking and cannot interpret the meaning of the things and actions she is watching with her eyes. But as the time passes, the child starts to learn the language of her parents and other members of her family. Slowly she starts to speak and learn new skills. This is a time when the light starts to appear in her mind as something in her mind opens up. With age as she learns new things and gains skills, her mind receives more light and fresh air. This is a simple concept of knowledge.

Our mind is a long infinite gallery with doors on both sides and is in complete darkness. As we open one door we get light and fresh air. Each of these doors is the door of knowledge. For example, one door can be of basic communication skills, while another door can be of fundamental physics or mathematics. As a person works hard to gain knowledge and develop skills, more doors in our minds are opened. The mind with more light and fresh air would have more confidence and have a higher probability of success in life.

You must have observed that the stammering reduces when we tend to speak in front of the child, as our knowledge and experience are much higher. The same is the case when we tend to speak in front of people who are much less skillful or knowledgeable than us. This is all because of relative confidence, which is due to relative light in mind. A person with more light would have more confidence, allowing her to communicate better.

As we know that confidence would be an essential element to defeat stammering. It means that if we can have more light and fresh air in our minds that would help us to defeat our stammering. That is what we have to do. We have to enhance our knowledge and develop skills and competencies to open more doors in our minds. More light would ensure stronger confidence and better communication.

Commit to putting extra efforts to develop your skills and improve your knowledge, definitely much more than people at par. You will be able to observe the difference in the coming weeks and months.

Speak with Pause

When you were a little kid in kindergarten, you learn to improve your handwriting through cursive writing practice. This workbook allowed you to write each letter slowly but written beautifully. It gave you guided lines to support you in your practice. In this exercise, we will perform the same activity, but instead of writing, we will speak. This practice would involve slow and controlled breathing and speaking each word with control.

Speaking with pause is considered to be one of the most powerful ways to deal with the stammering and defeat it. People have used it for decades and centuries with success. The objective of practicing this technique is simple. We have to consciously control our breath, thereby controlling the spoken word, one at a time. We will ensure not to rush through spoken words, instead, focus on every word giving it enough space to speak. This means speaking only a few words at a time while completing a few sets of words in one breath. We need to pause for a couple of seconds after every 2 to 3 words, before starting again. The pause should be long enough to have control over your breath and words. The pause could be around 2 to 4 seconds between the spoken words. This will allow your speaking organs to relax and release stress.

For example, if you have to speak a sentence with pauses in between (consider each comma as the pause for three seconds each). "I am, happy to see, your performance. I am sure, that you will, keep working, hard."

You can practice with different sentences every day for 10 to 15 minutes to have better control over your speech. Try it in your native language in addition to English. If this approach to speaking becomes a way of your speech then the control over your words will become better. Start using it immediately.

Speaking Tough Words with Rhythm

A person struggling with the problem of stammering would immediately find the ease in speaking when he starts to sing or recite a poem. It happens as singing allows words to slide on curves, instead of getting stuck in the sharp corners of normal speech. This can be understood by assuming to be traveling on the road with sharp curves at 90° in comparison to driving smoothly on a normal curvy road. The words tend to get stuck in the sharp corners but float smoothly on the curves. Songs and poems also have rhythmic words aiding the interrupted flow of words.

Speaking with curvy language is also considered impressive and sophisticated. Many top leaders, including several USA presidents, deliver their speeches in curvy language. Martin Luther King's speech "I have a dream" is one example.

We can use the concept of rhythmic words to speak tough words, which creates speaking difficulties. To use this technique, insert a rhythmic word, which can be easily spoken, before the difficult word. For example, if the difficult word is 'mommy', then the rhythmic words could be 'ommy' or 'hommy'. To speak 'mommy' in rhythm, speak the rhythmic word 'ommy' before it, in quick succession. So it would be spoken as 'ommy, mommy'. You can speak 'ommy' at a lower volume than 'mommy', so that only you listen to it. This technique will allow you to speak 'mommy' or any other difficult word smoothly.

Other examples are:

Difficult word- Khapa, Rhythmic Word- hapa or papa

Difficult word- Dilli, Rhythmic word- hilli or illi

Avoiding the First Letter of the Word

The difficulty of stammering start with a specific letter, which could be M, P, T or any other letter. This is common in every language. Once this specific letter in a word gets stuck, the person is unable to speak the word, and hence the whole sentence is delivered with interruptions. This situation raises anxiety levels which aggravate the problem of stammering. If you could solve this problem then we will be able to speak the specific word or this whole sentence. The best way to solve this problem is by avoiding speaking letters that are creating problems. For example, if the letter 'M' is creating the problem in 'mommy', then we can speak only 'ommy', after ignoring the letter 'M'. This way speaking the word and the sentence would be much easier with minimal stammering.

The question may arise that ignoring one letter would change the interpretation of the word, how to solve this problem? Our mind is a powerful and intelligent biological machine, which is capable enough to fill in the gaps by generating the required parts itself. The mind of the receiver of the word and sentence would fill in the missing letters, therefore getting the intended message. Most won't even notice any omission.

Other examples of this technique are:

Instead of 'Mummy' speak 'ammy' or 'hammy'

Instead of 'Papa' speak 'aapa'

Instead of 'Dilli' speak 'illi'

Message Communication with Different Words or Phrases

This is the most common technique used by the people who stammer. Generally, it is learned with experience, but it can be used effectively if we are consciously aware of it.

The subconscious mind triggers anxiety, whenever a difficult letter appears in our speech. We consciously know about it and have the fear of getting stuck in the word and sentence. The best way forward is to avoid that word altogether and express the same information or idea with different words in which the difficult word does not appear. That is the reason that occasionally we find some people speaking in long sentences with fogginess in their communication. We can find them going in circles without clearly and simply specifying the idea.

This technique comes with the trade-off between facing the trigger of stammering or communicating confusingly. As expected, people choose the latter. You can practice minimizing the confusion delivered in your communication with stronger word power and using better word combinations.

If this technique is used effectively then it can give immediate benefits of avoiding stammering altogether. Most people use it, some of them impressively. The best way to use this technique is to speak slowly and pause for a few seconds before speaking a sentence. It may look like that we are speaking artificially slow but with regular practice, it will become normal and more controlled. The pause between sentences would give us a chance to evaluate and avoid the difficult letters if present. The whole process will not take more than a fraction of second.

Some of the examples of this technique can be:

"I saw a big baboon" - This huge monkey was jumping and acting difficult.

"Sam is marvelous at meditation" - Sam is good at closing his eyes and focusing his attention on something, there's a word for this process, which I do not remember. But he is good at it.

This technique is used temporarily for immediate improvement in our speech and successfully communicating the message. As we are practicing with different exercises and techniques we will slowly get command over difficult letters and words.

Different Speaking Speeds

This technique is subconsciously* used in normal communication. While speaking at lower or higher than normal volume, we tend to speak slower than normal speed. While in anxiety, fear, frustration or anger, we speak faster than our normal speaking speed. The present technique will use this idea consciously.

The idea of this technique is to speak at different speaking speeds without changing your speaking volume. For example, while giving a speech or presentation we change our speaking speed to faster or slower than normal speaking speed. That is how we need to start practicing this technique.

To speak at a different speed than your normal speaking speed would require certain control in synchronization with different speaking organs. This can be a good exercise and practice for speaking. Professional speakers also practice using this technique. To add to the complexity of this technique, different speaking speeds can be random, without you expecting it. You can either use a digital application to present random numbers to you, with each number linked to a speaking speed. For example, 2- normal speed, 3- faster while 1- slower. If any application or software is not available then it can be outsourced to another person or you can do it yourself by randomly picking up a card with three numbers written on each.

To make this technique even more interesting and powerful, use five speeds instead of three. In this case, 3 will be the normal speaking speed, while 4- faster, 5- Very Fast and 2- Slower, 1- Very Slow.

You can practice this exercise once every day for 15 minutes.

This exercise is also excellent for improving the speech quality of everyone with the desire to speak better.

Precautions:

- The words must be spoken clearly to be understood by another person.
- Manage your breathing effectively during speech speed transitions.

**What is Subconscious-*

If your mind is an iceberg floating in the water, then its tip is the conscious mind, while the rest is the subconscious mind. It stores memories, experiences and emotions. Information stored in the subconscious becomes automatic and natural. For example, the driving skills of a vehicle are stored in the subconscious mind, which ensures minimal use of the conscious mind. The quality of life and performance of a person depends on the information stored in the subconscious mind. The habit of stammering also sits deep in the subconscious mind. To defeat stammering, your subconscious mind must be convinced of your abilities to speak well, without impediments. This can only be achieved with practice.

Lean a New Language and Speak it

Stammering is triggered by psychological fear due to the presence of a specific letter or word in the sentence to be spoken. This anxiety resides in your subconscious mind which is automatically activated, whenever that specific word is to be spoken. Since childhood, we speak our native language (mother tongue). The habit of stammering also started with this language. This habit is rigidly sitting in the subconscious mind for specific letters in the language. This pattern can be disturbed or even broken in a different language.

Learn a different language to weaken stammering. A new way to communicate will allow you to bypass the anxiety triggers that are activated in your local language. Your communication in a new language would have lesser impediments. Continuous practice with the new language would train your subconscious mind for your spoken fluency.

Use your new skill to interact with people in this language. This will be a good speaking practice, with reduced speech impediments. If possible, interact with native people to bring fluency and understanding to your language skills.

Self-Commentary

Speaking practice is necessary to improve your speaking and defeat stammering. Use the suggested exercises and techniques for speaking practice. It will be great if you can practice with other people like friends, family members and other interested people and groups. Many times, we are unable to find people or equipment to practice speaking.

Self-commentary is a technique that can be used anywhere, anytime and without the need for any person or tool. The material to practice self-commentary is also infinite. We understand the concept of commentary, a detailed audio description of an event such that any other person listening to it can visualize the described event and other hidden details.

In the technique of self-commentary, we will speak aloud about our actions and thoughts. These could be anything from commentary about making tea to polishing shoes. To expand the list of live speaking events, speak aloud the live commentary about other people and things. For example, you could be commenting about a man sitting on a bench in a park.

Self-commentary is a good speaking exercise. Practice speaking as much as you want. In addition to improving speaking skills, it will strengthen your command of the language used. For example, an individual learning German could present live commentary in the German language.

Use this technique to practice speaking skills for at least 40 minutes, every day.

Precautions:

- Speak optimally to not disturb others.

- Choose your location and speaking volume judiciously for privacy.
- Be rational while doing 'Self-Commentary' about others.
- Never encroach upon others' privacy.

Read Content Aloud

Constant speaking practice is a necessary element to defeat your stammering. The more you practice the better your confidence in speaking without impediments. You must find different opportunities to speak in various conditions and scenarios.

For getting more practice you can start reading any content aloud. While using this technique you must be careful that every word spoken must be clear, you should not be speaking any word casually. The objective is to train the subconscious mind so much that it believes your speech without impediments is normal, the way you speak. The acceptance of your normal speaking without stammering as truth, your speech impediments will reduce considerably and you can speak without much problem.

You need to be careful that your speaking aloud must not disturb anybody else. To start, practice alone without anyone in your vicinity. The volume of the spoken words should be around your normal speaking volume. You can practice speaking in your local language, English or any other language. Practice using this technique without tiring yourself or your speaking organs.

Please note that stammering is too rigid to be defeated easily. It would put a hard fight back. You must be ready to practice these techniques for the coming months and years, without visible drastic improvements. You must know that the improvement is constantly happening, which may not be visible initially, ensuring your victory in the war against stammering.

CHAPTER FOUR

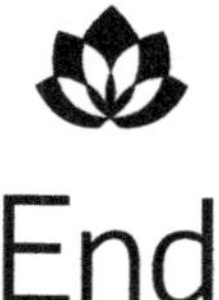

End

We did our best to present exhaustive information and powerful ideas to start and win your struggle in stammering. Remember stuttering is just a habit and it can be broken. You can win. This fight will take time, maybe many months to many years but in the end, you will be a transformed person and a good speaker.

Now you know everything to become an amazing speaker. Don't wait, commit and start with discipline and sincerity. Don't stop till you earn your right to speak freely, without the fear of words.

About Author

Anshuman is an author and knowledge creator who has transformed the lives and work of people from every continent. His groundbreaking ideas in Thinking, Communication, Personality and Storytelling are revolutionary, simple and effective.

His belief in simplicity has created powerful solutions that can be used by everyone effortlessly.

Experience the free material from following links:

https://direct.me/anshuman

About Ash #shorts

Ash #Shorts are the short, practical and simplified format of the complex ideas and topic that can be applied and utilized immediately.

9 798889 513612

Printed by Libri Plureos GmbH in Hamburg,
Germany